D1558069

Something Beautiful From God

Something Beautiful From God

Susan Schaeffer Macaulay

Cornerstone Books
Westchester, Illinois

Something Beautiful From God

Copyright © 1980 by Susan Schaeffer Macaulay
Published by Cornerstone Books
a division of Good News Publishers
Westchester, Illinois 60153

All rights reserved. No part of this publication, including the text, photography and design, may be reproduced in any manner, stored in retrieval system or transmitted in any form or by any means, electronic, mechanical, photocopy, recording, or otherwise, without the prior permission of the publisher, subject to the provisions of the United States copyright law.

Full color photography on front cover and pages 26, 28, 30, 32, 34, 36, 37, 41, 43, and 45 by Manus Huller from *Parents* magazine, October 1979. Property of *Parents* magazine, copyright © 1979. Used by permission through special arrangement.

All other photography (except page 76) property of Ron Seymour, copyright © 1980. Used by permission through special arrangement.

Book design by The Cioni Artworks

Printed in the United States of America

Library of Congress Catalog Card Number 80-67388

Clothbound edition: ISBN 0-89107-189-X
Paperback edition: ISBN 0-89107-186-5

Dedication

DEDICATION

This book is dedicated to a family

They'll know who they are

Three generations making a lot of noise

Usually cheerful

They make good friends

You'll know them if you happen

To bump into a crazy gang

Strolling, chattering, and enjoying each other

Next to a beautiful lake

In the early spring each year

Hi! Including the one who is at present

Amongst us, unborn but beautiful

Contents

Preface For Parents

"Where was I *before* I was born?"
"What did I look like?"
"What happens when a baby dies?"
"Why did God let Kathy be handicapped?"

Questions. Your child's face turned up expectantly. The answer you give or don't give will color that child's thinking for the rest of his or her life. You have the possibility of laying foundations now for an entire lifetime.

What do we offer our children? It is easy to give sugary-sweet answers. But will these stand the test of time? We owe our children truth. As Christians, believing the wonderful biblical answers, we can offer a sure hope based on sound reality.

I was privileged to grow up in L'Abri Fellowship, where from childhood on I was exposed to the exciting positive side of life. Through classical music and the fine arts we were shown how important beauty was to the human experience. Questions and their answers were also important. Then, while still a teenager, twenty-three years ago, I began regularly teaching children—from European, English, and American backgrounds—about the Bible and answering their many questions. Some were happily secure and some sad and disturbed. I discovered again and again that children respond to the truth about reality and are fascinated by factual knowledge as well. They are aware, too, of the sad side of life in an abnormal world—death, disease, sin. And they are comforted and secure in the knowledge that they don't have to be perfect before God will love them.

For the last nineteen years my husband, Ranald, and I have lived and worked in L'Abri Fellowship. Nine years ago the Lord gave L'Abri (French for "shelter") a lovely country home in England where approximately thirty students from all over the world come to study, question, and live for up to three months. By now we feel like grandparents to scores of new families! The varying questions and problems confronting these students have made me aware of the direction of thought in our society and consequently of the sorts of problems which children have to face as they grow up.

The greatest joy in my "work responsibilities" is being mother to four children aged between seven and eighteen years. Ranald and I have found that reading books aloud is a very important moment of our family day. Every evening, tired out from busy lives, we gather around a crackling fire. With hot drinks and fruit we all listen to Ranald reading a story. People and situations spring to life with his expressive reading. We laugh, wonder, are moved, and enjoy this half-hour best of all. It was therefore a natural step for me to write a book for families or schools that could be read aloud.

The beauty, wonder, and sheer excitement of the growing baby before birth is perhaps the most beautiful story that can be told. I have kept it a story of the baby's development—its worth and its beauty—from the first day of life (conception). I have tied in the positive side of eternal life as God has planned it. This is *not* a "sex education" book. Many important and beautiful facts before conception are outside of the scope of the first chapter. The last two chapters deal with special problems which relate to birth, families, and the handicapped child.

One of the questions I am often asked is how could I bring children into such a sad world. For me, the pure joy of giving birth to a dear and precious child is possible because of the sure promise of God in his Word that he has a solution for us through Jesus Christ. One need not be wrapped up in fear of the bad things that could be in store for the child. Each of us has the possibility of God's certain gift to us. Maybe this book will also encourage parents-to-be.

I have written about the miracle of development. I have not dealt with the destruction of life before birth or alluded to any willful act that would endanger a baby's life. All children, however, will sooner or later be confronted with this. Perhaps some will weep, as mine have. It is important that children *do* know about it before their teens. They need straightforward information. Perhaps you will take your family to see the film series, *Whatever Happened to the Human Race?* This deals with the worth of the person, the base upon which this worth is built, and practical questions about abortion, the aged, etc. I would advise you to read also my father's book, *Whatever Happened to the Human Race?*, if you wish a biblical, Christian perspective on many related questions. Before giving answers you need to have sorted them out!

My thanks go to everyone who has helped with this book. Thanks to my father and mother for their foundation-laying in my life, and thanks too for real answers to my questions. They also gave me the knowledge that caring for my own family was a top priority. (If you would like some excellent help with family life, I warmly recommend reading *What is a Family?* by Edith Schaeffer). Thanks to my brother, Franky, for without his encouragement I might never have started writing. Thanks too to the medical experts who checked up on the factual content of the manuscript. Thanks to Ray Cioni and Robbin Cadena for imagination in art directing and designing this book. But most of all, I am grateful to God, the giver of all life, and for his gift of his only Son. Thanks to him for life and not death, for light, truth, love, and beauty as found in his Word and in his creation.

Susan Schaeffer Macaulay

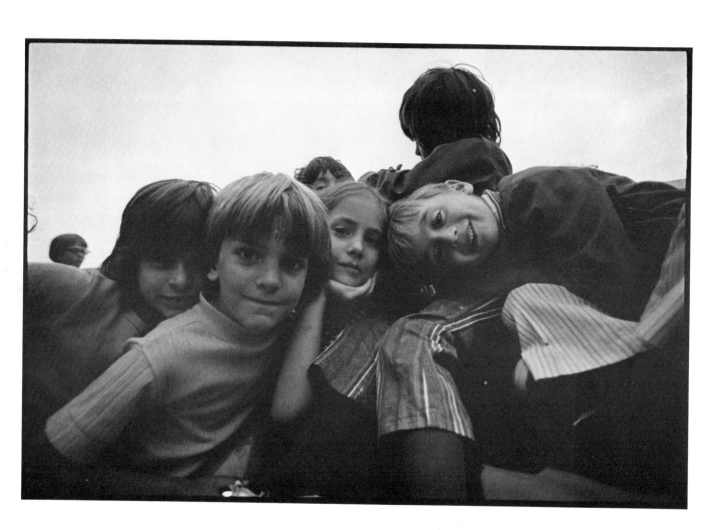

1

A Special Present: You

When did you begin to be *you*, different from anyone else in the whole wide world or even outer space? Was it on the day you were born? Of course, we all count our birthdays, whether we are three, nine, fourteen, or twenty-seven years old, from the day we were born. Your parents enjoy remembering that special day when they could at last look into your face and feel your tiny, warm body cuddled in their arms. At last the big answer to their question had come: it was a *girl* or it was a *boy*. They smiled and exclaimed, "Why, it was Mary all along!" Or, "I never knew it was John until today!"

Maybe your mother said, "He kicked so hard before he was born, I bet he's going to play football." She looked into your little crib and gently touched your head with a finger. "So *that's* the little head

13

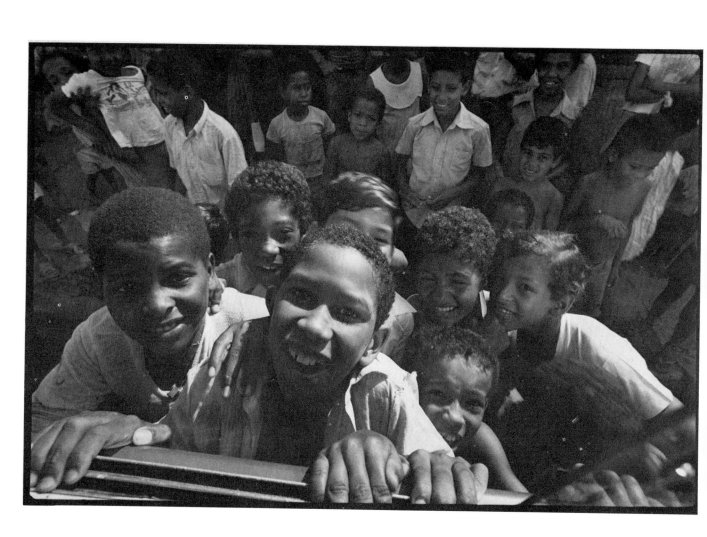

that I could feel in my tummy. Now I can see the little face of my very own baby.'' Maybe she laughed and said, ''My baby looks so tiny now; he seemed *such* a big load in my tummy.''

Your grandparents and uncles and aunts couldn't visit you fast enough. If they lived too far away, they wanted a photograph of you. Maybe your grandmother said, ''Oh, look at her ears. They are *just* like her Aunt Debby's.'' Or your grandfather said, ''He is so long and strong-looking. Our sons were all like that, too. He's a chip off the old block.''

Everybody was excited and happy. The birth of a new baby is one of the nicest things that can happen in a family's life. It is like Christmas morning. On Christmas morning we get to see and enjoy good things that may have been hidden in exciting, bumpy packages for weeks. On the day that you were born, your ''birth day,'' your family could at last see you.

But that wasn't when you began. You had been inside your mother for about nine months, all hidden away from sight. The family had guessed about you; now they could meet and name you. You were a very special present!

The very first day of your life, your ''life day,'' two little cells joined together. (Human cells are tiny parts of a man or woman, boy or girl; they are the building blocks of the human body. You are made up of many thousands of cells.) One egg cell was from your mother, and one sperm cell was from your father. This joining is called ''conception,'' or the

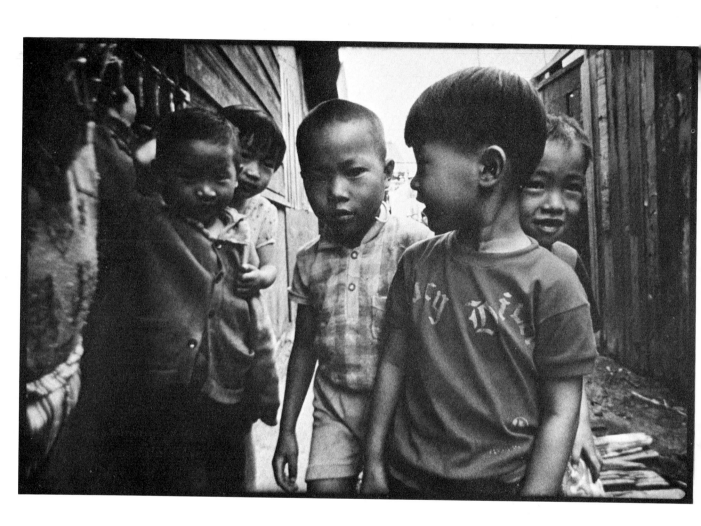

beginning of you as a separate individual. Just as a small acorn grows to become a huge oak tree, this tiny seed eventually became your body.

The mother's egg cell is so tiny that you could just about see it if you had the chance. Of course, we never do see an egg cell, because it is hidden in the mother's tummy. It would look like a very, very tiny dot. The father's sperm cell is so small that you would need a microscope to see it.

But even though these tiny cells can hardly be seen, they are made in a most amazing way. The cells have little tiny messages in them, the plans of the one person that can be born from them. Half of your plans came from your mother's cell, and half from your father's cell.

A few years ago, scientists discovered a chemical called DNA. This exists inside tiny threadlike bits in the middle of the cells. These bits are called chromo-somes, and they carry the tiny messages we were talking about. From your father's sperm cell came twenty-three chromosomes. From your mother's egg cell came twenty-three chromosomes. As soon as they joined, you had your first day of life! Your father's sperm cell made you a boy (a Y sperm) or a girl (an X sperm).

As soon as the two cells became one, the tiny cell that was you already had all the plans laid down to make you a different person from anyone else that is or who has ever been. Its chromosomes and the DNA stuff had the plans for your hair color, your skin

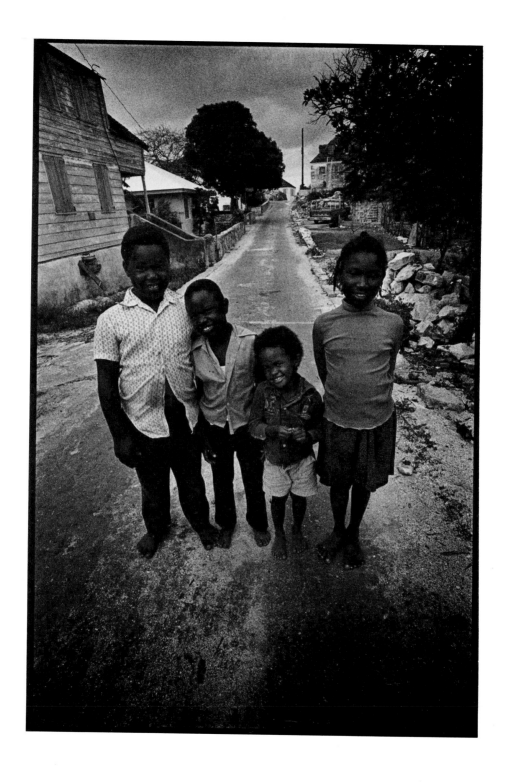

color, the color of your eyes, how tall you would grow, the shape of your nose. It also planned whether you would have the sort of body that could be good at running, or a mind that would be extra good at math. In fact, that tiny cell had thousands of messages. Only *you* could grow from it. (There is, though, an exception to this: identical twins. Such twins have exactly the same chromosomes and so are physically alike, though their personalities are probably very different.) Nevertheless, that cell was unique, and there is only one person who is you in the whole world.

Each time parents have another baby, the two cells that have come together have a different *arrangement* of plans. That is why brothers and sisters are different from each other. That is also why there are likenesses within a family. The plans come from your mother and father. They carry plans from your grandparents, too. That is important. You *belong* in your family.

As soon as the two cells joined to become one, the new cell started growing. The sperm had actually gone inside the egg and become part of it; this was now a fertilized egg. Your mother couldn't feel the fertilized egg settle into the wall of her womb or uterus, a safe place for the baby below her stomach. But her body was extremely busy doing all the right things to keep you safe, to help you grow. Those first secret days were very important ones in your life. You were so tiny and growing every minute.

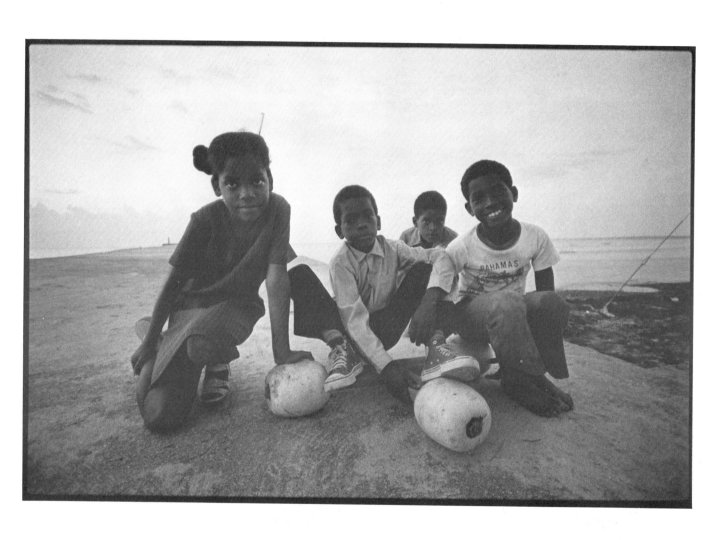

In those early days of your life, before anybody else knew you at all, when they didn't even know that you had started growing, someone knew all you about you. He knew your name, what you would look like, and what you would like to do. This was God. He knows everything. He had made everything in the first place. He loved you already. You were very, very precious to him, and he cared about you. He is interested in babies because he loves every person.

Even before you were born, the Lord God had already given you a gift. He knew that the world was spoiled after Adam and Eve had chosen to sin, to disobey him so long ago. He knew that you would do wrong things, too, when you were old enough.

And he knew that you would have to die sometime. But God cared for you before you were old enough to think about him or to choose anything for yourself. God's gift for you was waiting for the day when you could understand about how he had loved you. On that day, you would be able to say, "How *wonderful!* Now I see that God sent his only Son, Jesus, because he loves *me*. Now that I believe in him, he has promised he will forgive me my sins and give me everlasting life."

Think of the beautiful plan that God had for you, as you were only just starting to grow! God wanted the best for your whole life, including the time when he has promised that we can live forever. As your life started, the giver of all life, God, cared all about you.

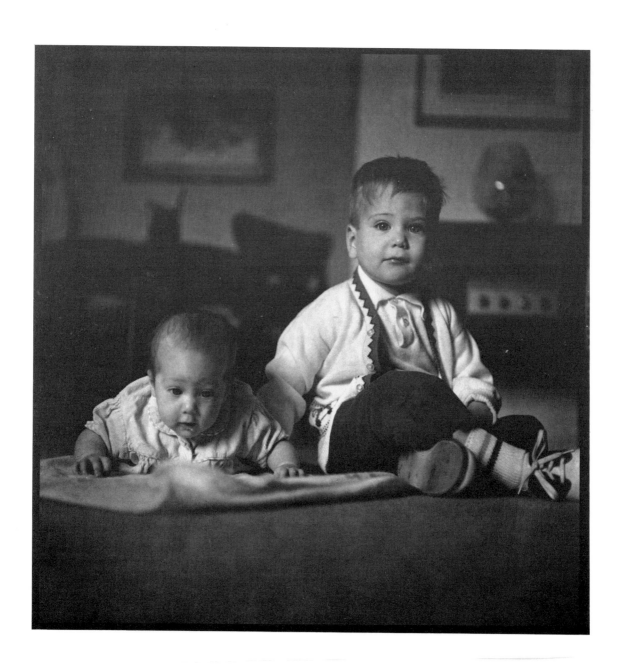

You sure didn't know all that in the first days of your life! But God knew all about it. He knew that when you were finally born you would be born into a world where Jesus had already come. He had already given a gift of life *forever* for you. So, as God saw you growing as a baby, he had a plan that you could become his very own child and have your sins forgiven.

Even when you were *so tiny,* an unborn baby, you had quite a future ahead! God has promised us life forever in heaven if we believe in him.

Your Creator, God himself, had a truly wonderful plan for you, the tiny baby—you who were already different from any other person. He wanted to be best friends with *you.* He loved you and he wanted you to love him back. He wanted you to talk to him and to understand his Word, the Bible. He made the beach for you to enjoy. He made the hills beautiful for your eyes when you go hiking, or camp, or have picnics. He made you so that you would enjoy painting nice pictures and would have fun singing or dancing to music. He made you so that you would race around and have quiet times with your very own friends. He made you so that you could think of good ideas and do them.

Our Lord God is our Creator and our King. He is the most important person in the whole world or in outer space. And in those first days of your life, he was the only one who knew *all* about you, and he loved you.

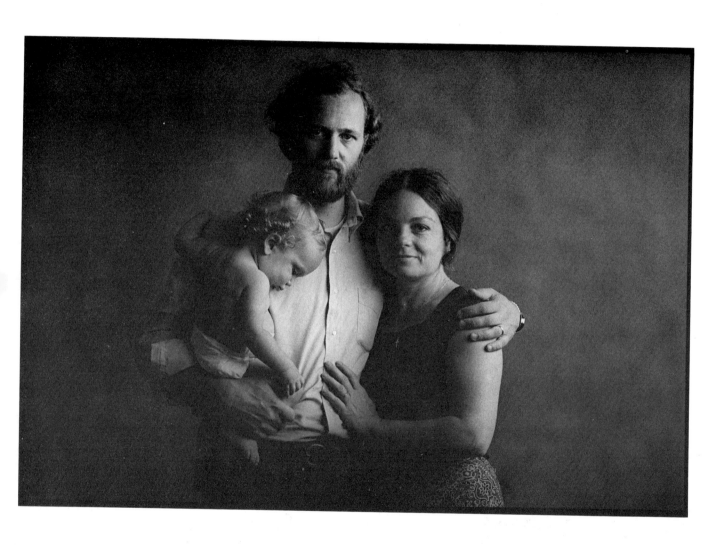

2
Every Day Something New

By the time your mother and father knew your life had begun, you were safe and secure in the womb in your mother's body.

Four weeks after your life day (conception), were you still an egg cell? Oh no! You were growing faster then than you will ever grow again. It is like a miracle to see how perfectly you were turning into the baby that the cell had started. You had your head, and your eyes, ears, mouth, and brain had started forming. Your little heart was beating away. You were very much alive! You also had the beginnings of your digestive tract; that is where all your food goes when you eat.

Every cell that makes up the tiny baby is a human cell, with just the right number of chromosomes for a *human* baby. And as we saw before, you were made

25

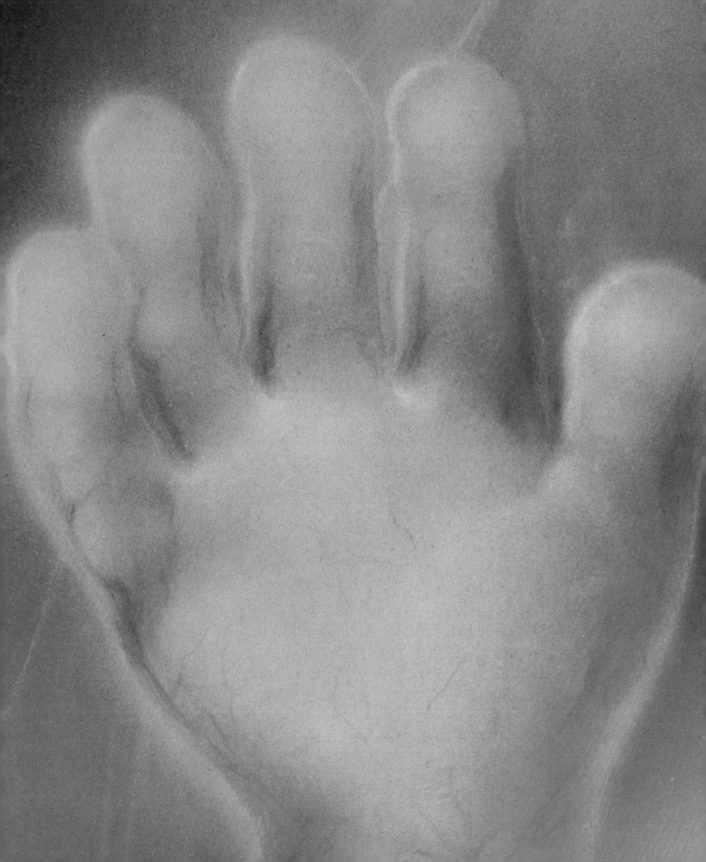

up from your very own parents' cells. You were already you!

In the second month that you were growing, new bits of yourself developed every day. It was as if you were the bud of a flower. You had first a bud in each place where an arm or leg would grow. Meanwhile, your brain took shape. Then your arms grew out, and on another day chubby hands grew.

How did God plan for the hidden you to be looked after? Well, the mother's body stretches to hold her growing baby. Even if the mother doesn't know yet what is happening in her womb, her body goes right ahead and cares for the baby. Like all living persons, the unborn baby needs good food to eat and air to breathe. But the baby can't eat with its mouth or breathe with its nose like we do. Instead, the mother's blood carries specially prepared food and air into her womb. The food and air then travel to the baby through the umbilical cord, a tube going from the mother's womb to the baby's bellybutton (its real name is ''navel'').

That amazing system not only brings in the *good* things the baby needs, but gets rid of all the wastes. The mother's blood carries the waste away. The baby's blood never mixes with the mother's blood. Your blood did its own job. Your tiny heart pumped it around your tiny body.

A bag of fluid or liquid forms around the baby to keep it safe. The baby floats in warm water in a protective bag. That way, the baby is comfortable

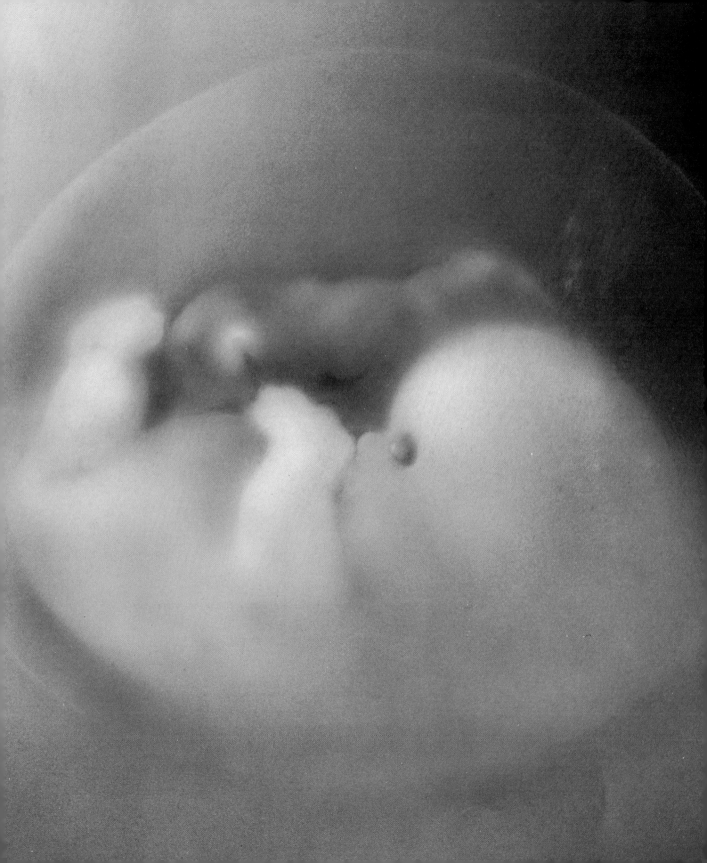

and safe from bumps and knocks.

The picture shows what you looked like after seven weeks.

That was what happened to you in the seven weeks after the two cells met and you began your life.

Of course, you were too young to be born. You were only about an inch long. You couldn't breathe or eat by yourself yet. Though your mother now knew that she was going to have a baby, you were so tiny she was still wearing her usual clothes. Her tummy still hadn't stretched too big. Maybe she went to the doctor for the first time. He examined her and said, "Oh yes, you *are* expecting a baby." Maybe your mother kept it a secret for another month, sharing it just with your dad. They already thought about the baby who would be big enough to be born in seven months' time. Or maybe your mother was the bouncy, excited sort of person. Maybe she telephoned *her* mother and sisters or friends the minute she knew. "Guess what? We are having a *baby*. Yes, I'm sure now!" she said.

Your mother knew that she could take good care of you, even though she couldn't see you yet. She drank more milk, and ate eggs, meat, and wheat germ. She knew that her tiny baby was at an important stage, and that you needed good food to grow strong bones, teeth, and muscles. She ate vegetables and oranges so that you would have plenty of vitamins. That helped *her* body, also. It is quite hard work for a mother's body to make a whole, healthy baby!

29

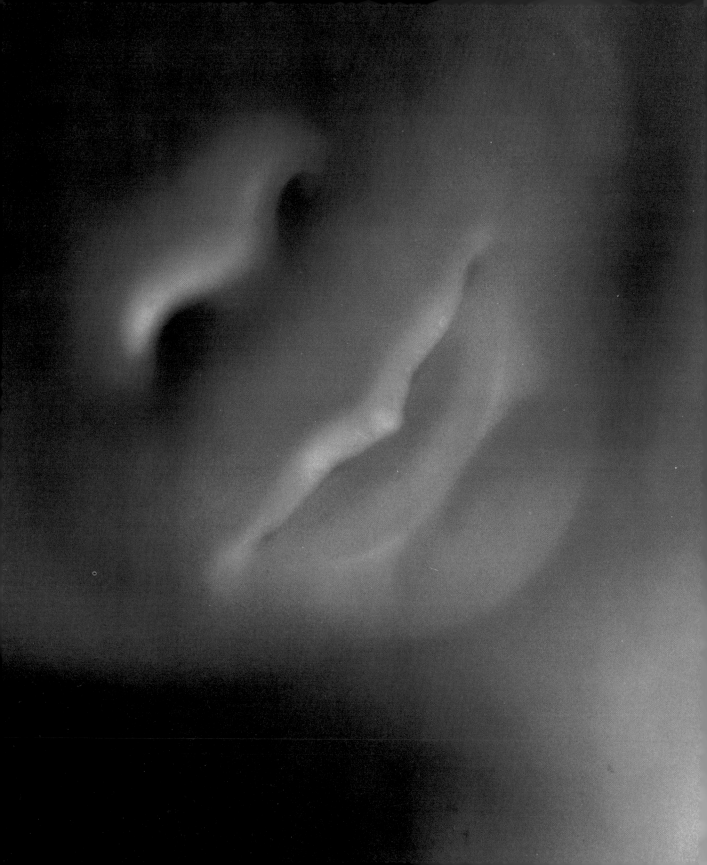

Your dad helped you grow safely, too. He helped your mother in different ways; for instance, by making home pleasant for her and the family. He thought a lot about you, and he was excited that he was going to have his own son or daughter. Maybe he worried about you. Maybe he said to your mother, "Now don't eat or drink anything that could hurt our tiny baby."

You were only eight weeks old, but other people were already taking care of you. (And, of course, God was watching over your growth.) Your mother wanted help from people who knew more about growing babies than she did. From the time that she was sure that you were there until your birth, doctors and nurses checked her and you every few weeks to see that you were both all right.

Sometimes people ask, But was I really a person then? Didn't I just look like a funny doll? Did it matter so much about what happened to me? Well, what happened to the safety of your life then mattered just as much as it would later on when you would be born and afterward. Have you seen a newborn baby? If it was a girl, she didn't look like she will when she is a grown-up. She didn't *act* like she will when she is twelve years old. But she was still a person; in other words, she was already an *individual* with her own body, feelings, and thoughts—and even her own likes and dislikes.

By the time your parents were sure that you were growing, your same body that you have today was

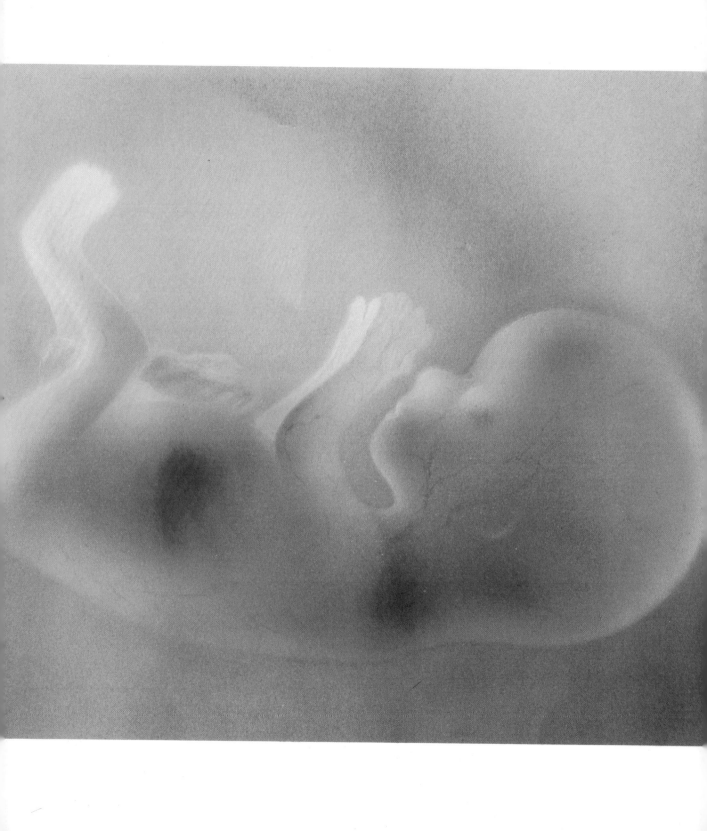

already formed and working. It was the same brain, the same heart, the same head. Every day you looked more and more like the newborn baby that you would be. And after you were born, this growth kept up. Even though the changes are not as obvious now, every day you look more and more like the grown-up you will be. Every day you learn how to do new things.

All along, from the time the two cells join and start out on the adventure of human life, it is the same individual, and will be for ever and ever. We know that only God gives life. We thank him every time a new life starts. We know that he doesn't love us only if we grow up to be strong or clever or good. He loves us even if we are weak and poor. He has especially told us to protect and care for those who are. That is why we must all take good care of babies, even when they are so tiny that they cannot live away from the mother or do anything to help themselves, even before they are born.

Now we are up to what had happened to you by the time you were twelve weeks old; that is about three months after your life day, your beginning or conception. By now you had become quite active! If you win a race at school now or ski nicely or swim well, you should remember that you started your practicing when you were not yet twelve weeks old. You were only about three inches long and you only weighed about one ounce.

You kicked away, but you were so tiny that prob-

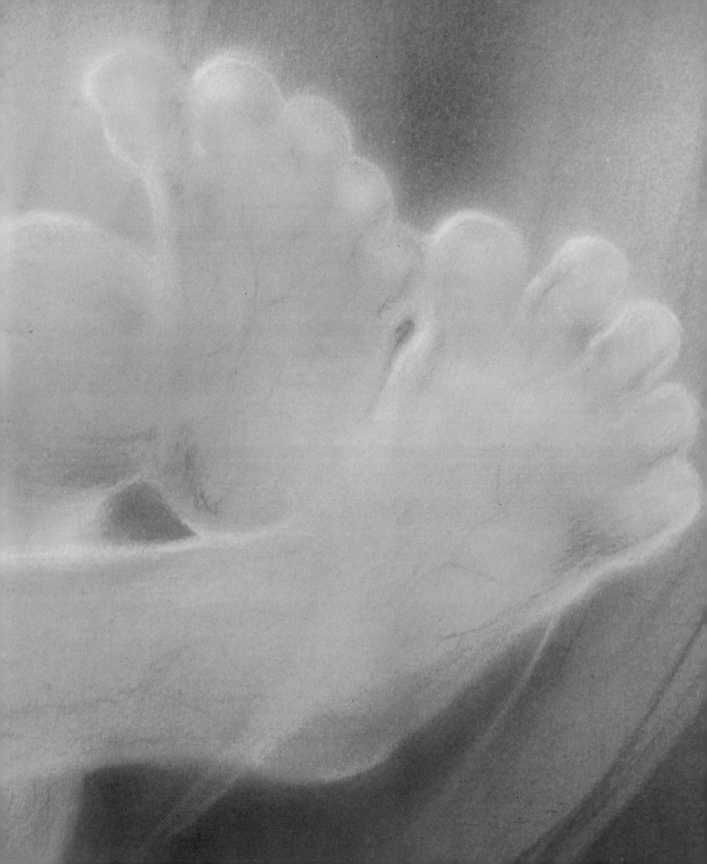

ably your mother couldn't feel it yet. You could turn your feet (good for skateboard practice). You could make a fist. You could move your thumb and bend your wrist. It would have been fun to peek at your tiny face! You turned your head around; you frowned, squinted, and opened your mouth. Actually you were pretty good at all these new activities, because you had been doing a bit more every day.

Your little fingernails started to grow. Your body already showed evidence of being either a girl's or a boy's. It seems amazing, but if you were a little girl you already had some egg cells for when *you* would grow up, so that *you* could have babies. And you were only three inches long! If you were a boy, you had some sperm cells in you so that someday *you* could be a father!

You were getting ready to be able to eat. Your lips were formed, and your whole mouth and cheeks started getting ready for sucking.

This particular month, the third month after your life day, was as important a one for you as you'll ever have.

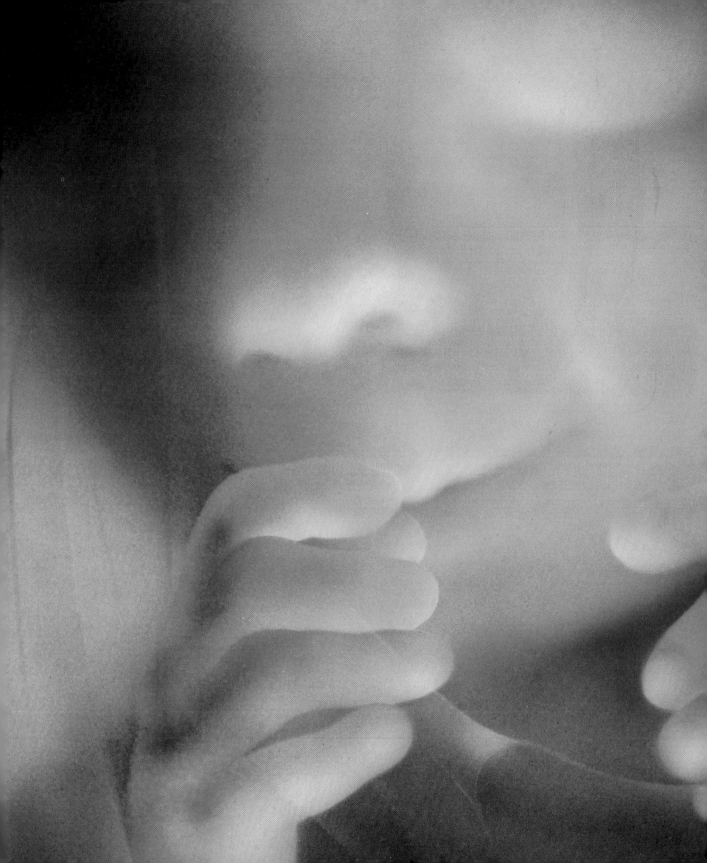

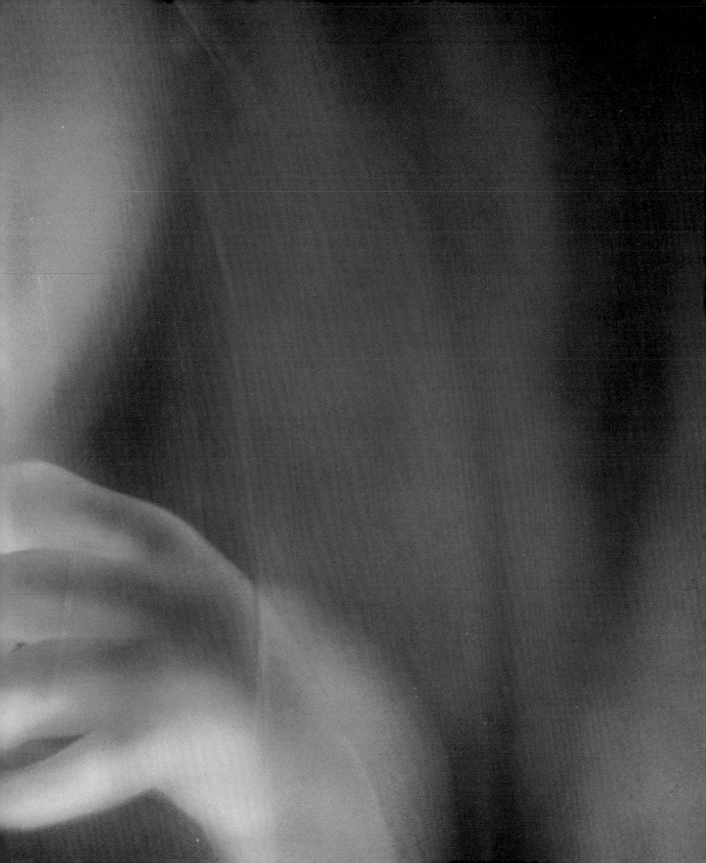

3
Nearly Finished

You know now that those weeks when nobody could see you, while you were growing inside your mother, were about the most important weeks in your whole life—even though you were so small that your mother was still wearing her ordinary clothes, although her jeans were probably tight! Inside, you grew on, wriggling, moving, and doing things. Then one day, when you were about six or seven inches long, when you weighed a bit less than a pound, your mother felt you kicking! You had been in her tummy about four and a half months. You were halfway to your birth day.

That first time, your mother wasn't sure if what she felt was you moving inside her. Was it . . . ? she wondered. She was excited. Until now, she could only *think* about you. Mothers think a lot about their tiny growing babies. Maybe she had started knitting something for you. Maybe your dad had already planned to hike with you on his back in just a few more months. In one or two days, your mother was *sure* that it was you kicking. Every time she felt you, it made her happy. Soon she would even get worried if you didn't kick. ''Oh,'' she might say, ''my baby is so quiet today; I hope it's okay!''

At first your kicks only made tiny fluttery feelings. It pleased your mother to realize how quickly you were getting bigger. Every day she felt stronger thumps. You were actually doing a lot more than just thumping around, including going to sleep and waking up. When you slept, you would even choose a position you found comfortable. Some babies curl up to sleep and some stretch out more. By the time you would be born, you would already have your own sleeping habits. When did you get a favorite position? In the womb!

So you now not only looked different from other babies of this age, but you acted differently too. Maybe your mother found that when she lay down after rushing around all day, you would choose *that* time to wake up and get active. Some doctors think that is why newborn babies tend to be wakeful in the evenings. They are used to being awake and kicking at that time!

As you got bigger, sometimes your mother would feel a dear little round bump pushing against her tummy. She sometimes pushed you back and felt you

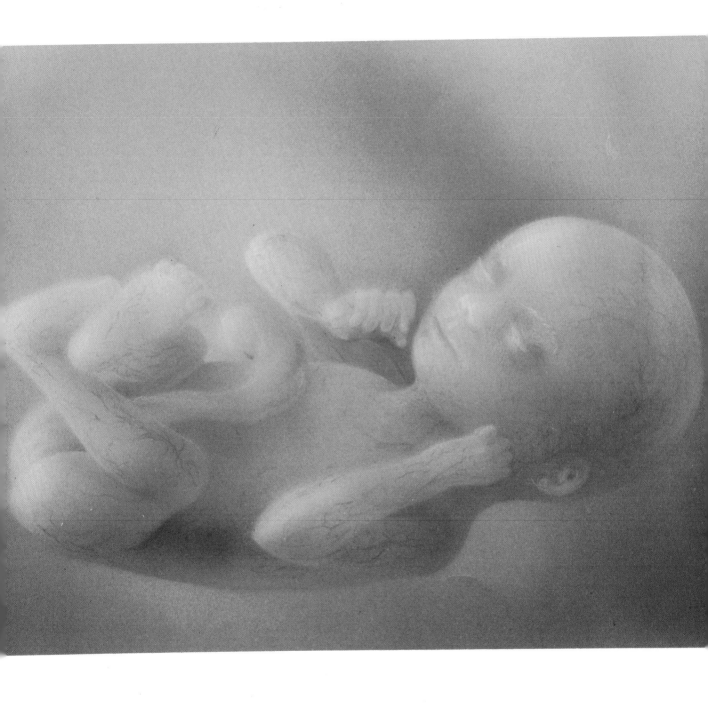

move away. Or sometimes she would put her hand over her tummy and pat you! ''I wonder if that is my baby's head or its little round bottom.'' When you had grown really big, your dad could see your tiny feet and hands moving like little lumps across your mother's tummy. He could *feel* you go thumpety-bump. You would turn somersaults until you grew so big that there was no more room. You were all safe and cozy. You could do whatever you felt like doing.

You had finished being formed in the first weeks of your life before birth. Now you were not only getting bigger day by day, but a few last beauty touches were added. Your eyebrows and eyelashes were formed at six months. Your head was no longer way too big for your body. Your fingers opened and closed and you could have held things if they had come into your hand. Your eyes opened, and they could look all around. Of course, there was nothing to see yet, but you were all ready for the big day! You could hear music, though, as sound came into the womb! Babies tend to wake up and kick a lot when they hear music. Was that your first dance? You heard your mother's heart day and night. If everything was rocking away quietly and you were sleeping, and then your mother dropped some pans with a crash, you would jump and wake up.

Sometimes you would get hiccups. You would jerk and shake with them. Your mother would feel you hiccuping away! The doctor could hear your heart too. He could listen to your heart with a stethoscope

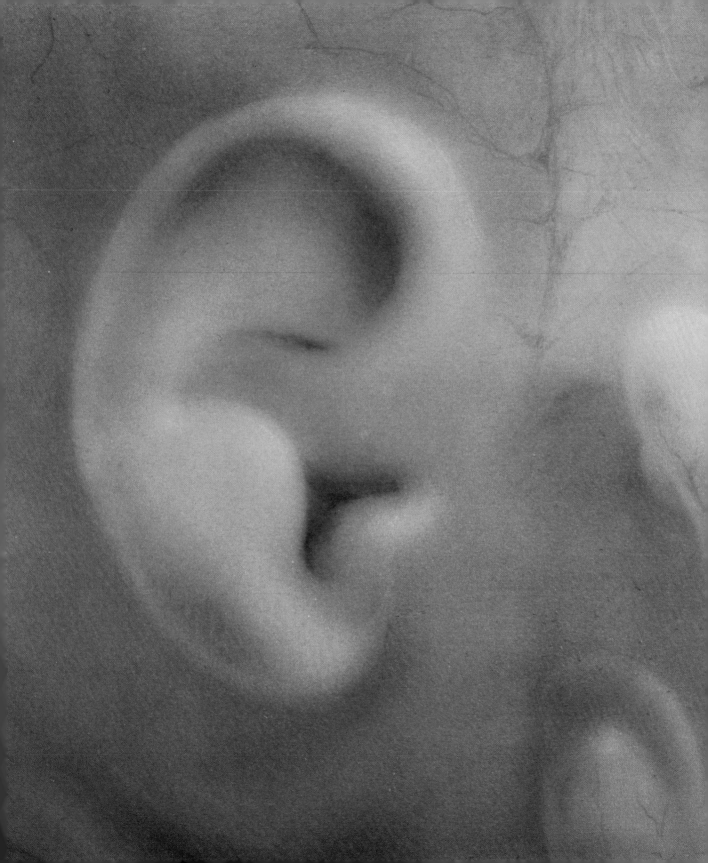

that he would put on your mother's tummy when he examined her. That way he knew that you were healthy. He said to your mother, ''The heart is beating strongly.'' That made her happy. She would tell your dad that night.

By the time you had been growing twenty-four weeks, or six months, you were really quite strong. If you had been born then, you would have had a chance of being able to live with special care in a hospital. The problem is, such tiny babies have trouble breathing. After all, God designed it so that nine months in the mother's womb is best. (A baby who is born early is called ''premature.'')

I know about a little girl who was born when she was only thirty weeks old. Her parents were worried that she would die, but she lived!

A baby born at this age first of all has to start breathing, and then keep on breathing if it is going to live. The baby hasn't yet put on enough fat to keep warm, so it has to be in a very warm place. A mother's womb is about ninety-seven degrees. That is like a hot, hot day in summer.

Clever people invented a warm bed to care for tiny babies. It is called an incubator. The air can have extra oxygen added, to help the baby breathe better. The bigger the baby is when it is born, the more chance it has of living. The premature baby is too tiny to suck milk from its mother's breast or from a bottle. So a tube like a thin, soft straw is slid into its tummy. Carefully a special nurse feeds the tiny baby.

44

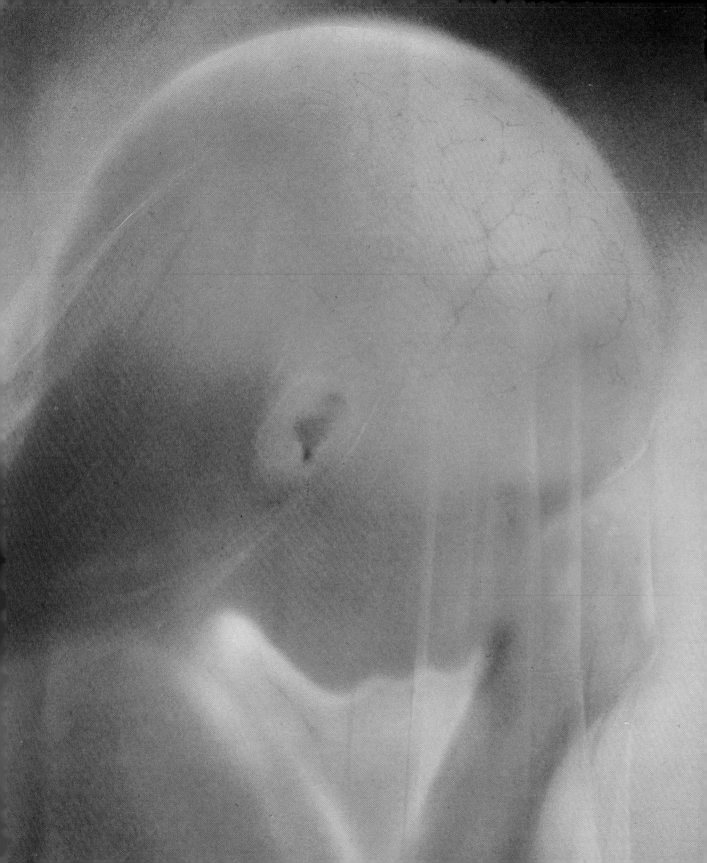

She pours liquid into the tube. She makes sure that the baby is breathing all right. The baby is too weak to be lifted, but the nurse cares for him right there on the tiny, warm bed. She slips a clean diaper under its bottom without pinning it on, because she doesn't want to bother the baby.

The nurses caring for these babies have to watch out that cold and flu germs don't come into the special nursery. Nobody comes into the room unless he has to. The mothers and fathers are allowed to visit their baby. They can touch the tiny arms and stroke the little cheeks. They love their baby. When possible, they are allowed to hold the baby in their arms. They are thankful that hospitals have special care nurseries.

I hope that your mother was able to carry you in her womb nine months.

Maybe some of you reading this did start off having special care. I guess that you are pretty thankful that you had that extra help! Your parents were so relieved the day that you were healthy enough to leave the hospital and come home.

What happens if a tiny baby dies before it is born, at any number of days or weeks? Or what if the baby is born, but never breathes?

If this happens, we are truly sad. We know that a person has died. The baby is never only a piece of the mother and father that just gets thrown out. Remember, from the very first day, its life day, the baby had its own self, different from any other person in the

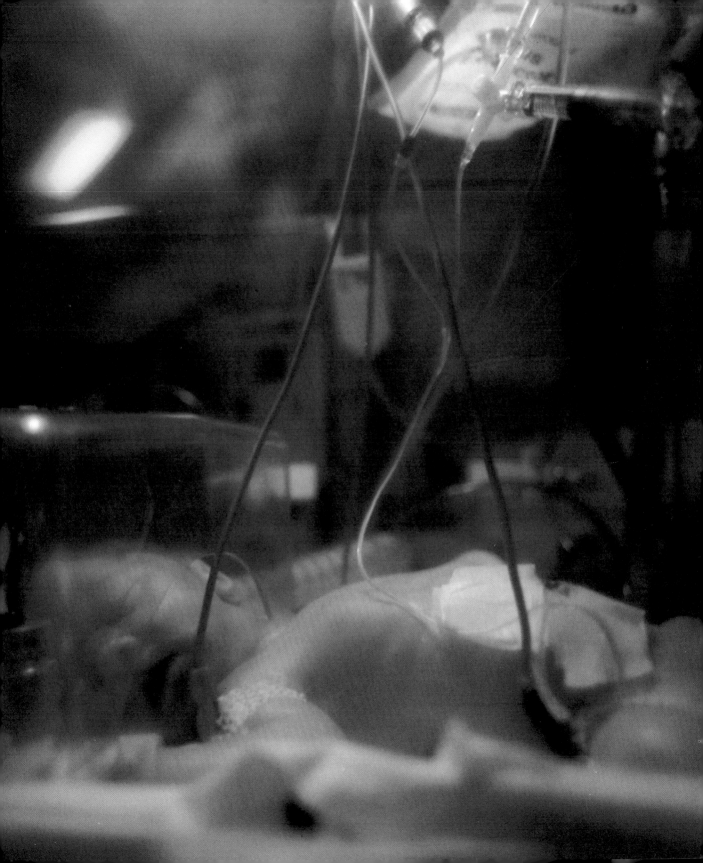

world. Remember that God cares about that person and loves each child. He doesn't love us because we are clever, strong, perfect, or only when we get to be grown-ups. He loves *us*. Jesus said, "Don't ever stop little children from coming to me, I love them." He also said that the Lord God Almighty even sees each sparrow that dies. Then Jesus said, "And aren't *you* worth a lot more than a sparrow?" Such helpless tiny babies who grow unseen to us are seen all along by our Lord God, and they are important to him. He loves each person.

Because of his great love, tiny babies who die go to Heaven. One day the child will be raised from the dead and will have a body that will never get sick or die.

I know a mother who has three children growing up. But she had five babies. Two died, at different times, before they were born. The parents wept with sorrow. They had wanted their babies to live! It seemed all wrong. But then, as they were comforted, they remembered that in Heaven they would meet their other two children. The mother says, "I have had five children, but only three are alive on earth. I am waiting to meet the other two in Heaven."

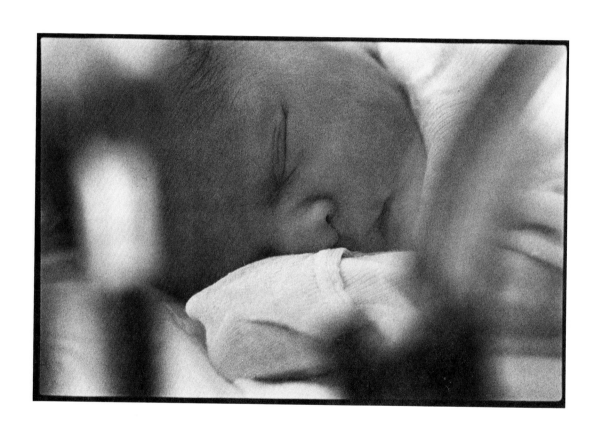

4 Your Birth Day!

We have come to the last weeks of your story, before you were born. You were putting on weight fast. Hair grew on your head, and you practiced sucking. Maybe you were one of the babies who sucked your thumb before you were born!

You didn't jump around as much. You had grown so big that the womb was a bit tight around you. Your head probably stayed lower than the rest of your body, waiting to be born.

You were ready to live in the outside world. You had a nice chubbiness, so that you could keep warm in ordinary room temperature. You were ready to suck milk, swallow, and digest it. You could see, hear, and feel. You were ready for the first gasp of breath and ready to breathe without any special help.

Your mother couldn't wait for you to be born! You were

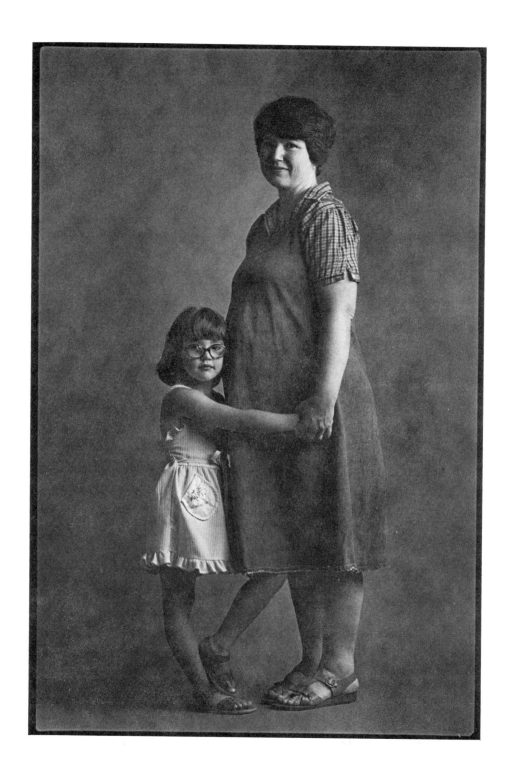

pretty heavy to carry around, and it felt uncomfortable. Maybe her back or legs ached by the end of each day. She probably had been getting ready for your birth. She had prepared your tiny shirts, diapers, a little bed, and other things you would need. If you had older brothers or sisters, they sometimes wished that you would be born soon too. Your dad felt this time was a special time for him. All along, you were his own baby. Soon he would hold you in his arms. Soon you would be with your family.

One day, or night, your mother felt her tummy muscles tightening. Again and again she felt this tightening (called contractions or "labor pains") as her womb began to open to let you out. This was your birth day. I cannot tell you exactly what happened on your birth day. I do know that your mother was excited and happy. At last your parents would be able to see you. Were you a girl or a boy? This was a big day for them! They probably went to the hospital for your birth. It usually takes several hours for a baby to be born. First of all, the cervix (sort of a fleshy plug in the womb) has to open, to let the baby's head push out. Special muscles do that, and it can take a long time. Your mother and father probably talked and read while they were waiting. If the pulling made your mother's back ache, maybe your father rubbed her back and helped her settle in a more comfortable position.

"It won't be long now," the doctor said.

Maybe your mother was then wheeled into a spe-

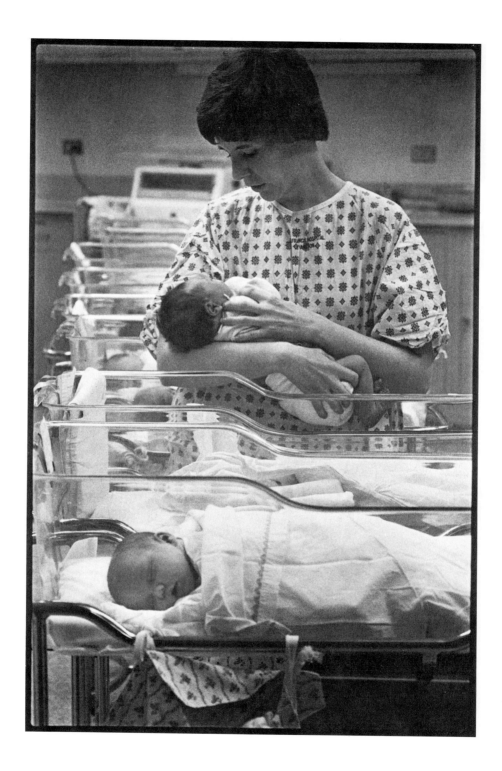

cial room where babies are born. Everything is there that might be needed to help a mother and her baby. Dads often come in to be near. It is exciting and beautiful to see a dear little baby being born. The dad is helpful. He can help the mother get propped up, so that it is easier for her to make her muscles push the baby out. This is hard work for the mother. (Of course, the doctor does quite a bit to help the baby come out, too.)

The baby's head starts pushing down with each contraction. The mother feels like pushing hard. She pushes, and the baby moves a little at a time down a special passage from the womb to the opening between her legs. This passage is called the vagina. The vagina stretches all around the baby's head. The mother keeps pushing to help her baby to be born.

"Oh!" the dad says, "I see its head now!"

The mother doesn't push too hard while the baby's head is being born. In another minute, the baby slides out. Maybe you were already crying on your birth day. You were all blue when you were born, but as you cried you turned a lovely pink all over.

Your mother smiled. A girl! Or a boy! My baby!

You were wrapped in a warm towel. Since you didn't need to be linked to your mother anymore, the doctor cut the umbilical cord. This didn't hurt. You breathed all alone.

Maybe your mother reached out her arms. Maybe she held you and kissed your beautiful head. Maybe your father walked around with you in his arms and

55

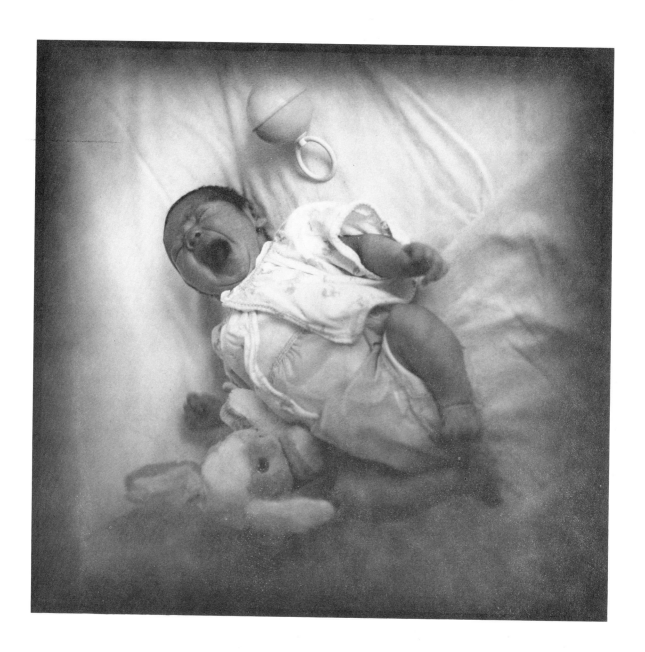

had the happiest smile on his face that he had ever smiled. Maybe you cried and your mother let you suck milk from her breast. Maybe you snuggled right down and loved it!

But I can't tell you exactly, because things start happening differently after we are born.

Each birth is different. And from then on, you had your own life to live, and it was different from anyone else's. But in these chapters I have tried to tell you what happened in the first 266 days of your life.

All babies are persons. You were different from a little animal baby. Because you are a person, you think about things, do things, and choose. You do good and bad things, silly things and important things. You love some people. You have friends. Sometimes everything is fun and easy; other times are hard for you. You are a person!

You are special; there is only one you! On that day when you were born, your family was thrilled to have you with them at last. They gave you your name, and they loved you.

Remember, too, that God loved you, and had planned a way for you to have your sins forgiven, become his special child, and receive everlasting life. But this plan depends on *you*. Did you know that? You couldn't say yes or no about whether or not you would be born. But God lets you choose whether or not you will be *his* child. For his plan to work out, you need to say, "Yes, I thank you for Jesus. I believe that he is God's Son, and that he came to take the punishment for my sin. Thank you.''

It is good to have life! And it is real life to know that we are God's children and will live forever and ever! It's fun to enjoy the world around us. It's good to know that we will live in a perfect world one day where nothing will go wrong again.

Your birth day was an important day in your life. An even more important day was the one, nine months before, when you started life at conception. But on your first day of birth, you were only interested in snuggling down in your mother's arms, and finding the sweet warm milk just for you.

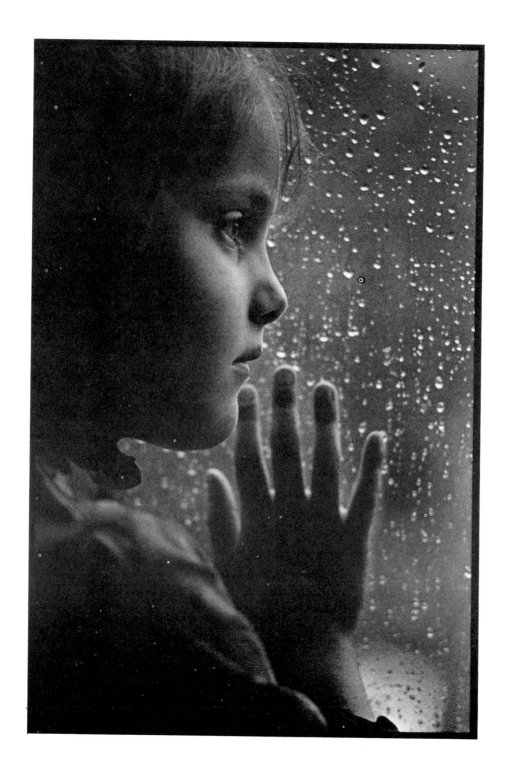

5
Extra Help Needed

When you plan something, it sometimes goes wrong, doesn't it? Like the day it rained and spoiled the special picnic party. Sometimes really big important things go wrong, and we need help badly. In the same way, different things can make it hard or dangerous for the mother and the tiny unborn baby she is carrying in her womb. Such people need our help in different ways.

For instance, some mothers do not have enough money to buy the good food they need if the baby is to grow strong and well. We can help buy food for them. I know some Christians who were worried about little African babies whose mothers never seemed to have enough food. They thought and prayed about it. They told other Christian people about the need. These people then gave money. Some

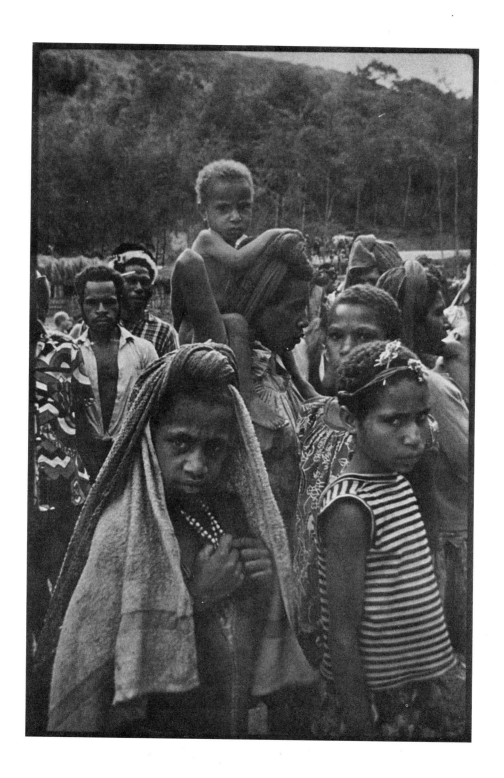

nurses and doctors said that they would give up their jobs and go to Africa. A young Christian farmer and a man who was good at building also went to help.

They went to a place where for miles and miles people hadn't had enough food to eat. The builder built a small clinic. The nurses and doctors soon had lots of people coming to them. Their special job was to care for little children who were hungry. They explained to the mothers that the children needed more milk and other good food. Christians had given big bags of good cereal that had lots of protein in it. But the nurses didn't only help the children who had been born. They tried hard to help mothers who were carrying tiny babies in their wombs. By giving the mothers the right foods, they helped the mother *and* the baby.

While the people at the clinic were doing this, the farmer was busy too. He went to the schools and helped boys and girls grow good vegetables to eat. He sold the farmers a kind of goat that gives more milk. He taught them how to grow good crops. Soon *everyone* was doing better in that valley. The babies who were born were healthier because of the good care.

Mothers and their unborn babies need all kinds of help. Some mothers are all alone. Some have had their husbands leave them. Some don't have enough money. A lonely person needs good friends. Maybe the mother doesn't even have a home. She feels frightened. She thinks, "I won't be able to care for

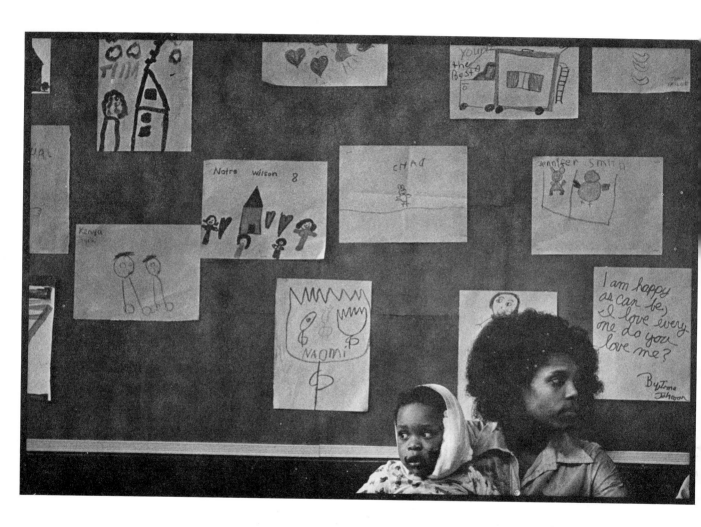

this baby by myself."

A girl named Jane was like that. I am sad to say that the daddy of the baby had just gone away and left Jane and her unborn baby. Jane was frightened because she didn't have much money or a home. "What will happen to my baby?" she wondered. "I don't want a baby right now!"

A friend of Jane's, called Di, asked Jane why she was so sad. Di gave Jane a hug, and then made her a good supper. She helped Jane by listening to everything, and then she talked to her. Di said, "You won't be all alone, Jane. I believe in God, and he loves you a lot. You can find out all about the Lord's care. I'm glad that I can be your friend. Why don't you come live in my apartment? I have just started looking for someone who could share my rooms here. The first thing you need is a home."

Di helped Jane by listening to her fears and by helping care for Jane's needs. She helped Jane find a job to earn money until the baby was born. They had good times too, and they had fun planning for the little baby who was going to be born. At last Jane came to that exciting day of birth. Even though at first she had felt badly about being pregnant when she hadn't planned it, now she was not only used to the idea of having a baby, but thrilled when the nurse said, "It is a boy, and he is healthy."

"Oh," breathed Jane, "he is beautiful! Look at his tiny hands! I love him."

Of course, everything was not completely easy for

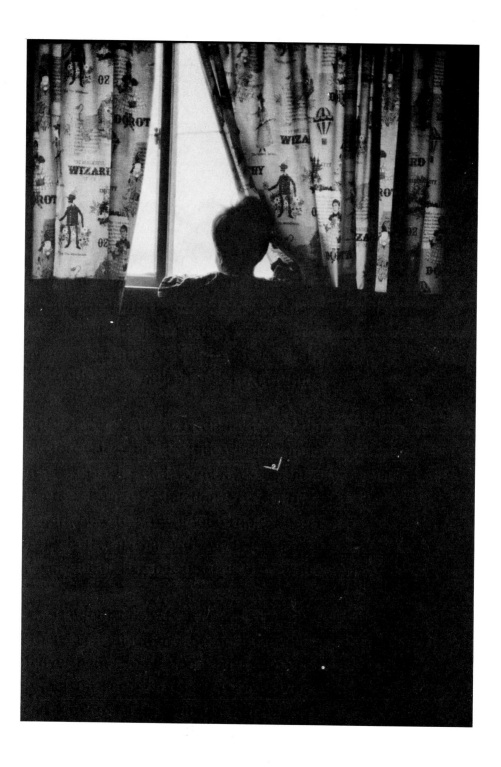

Jane and her tiny baby. This work sometimes *is* hard. However, the Lord had helped Jane through a good friend, Di, and he would not leave her alone now.

Most babies are born to a family where they are eagerly expected. However, sometimes when women find out that they are pregnant, it *is* hard for them. They are the ones who need our special help, friendship, and prayers. And by helping the mothers, we help those tiny babies who cannot help themselves. Jesus said that we are to help the weak, the poor, the helpless. That is what an unborn baby is. This is not only something that is nice to do; it is something that we *must* do if we obey Jesus.

Often, if mothers are given the right kind of extra help when things are hard, they can get over the hard time. People may find the jobs or homes they need or get better after being sick. Lonely people sometimes find someone who loves them, and they get married and have a family.

Something special sometimes happens for little babies if, after they are born, their mother can't take care of them. Maybe the mother has even died. Another family can choose to adopt the baby. The family may be a husband and wife who have longed for a baby, but no baby ever came. Or maybe it is a family that already has some children in it. These people say, ''We choose this one baby. We want it to be a member of our family.''

I will tell you about Sally and Ted. When Sally was a little girl, she loved to play with her dolls. She

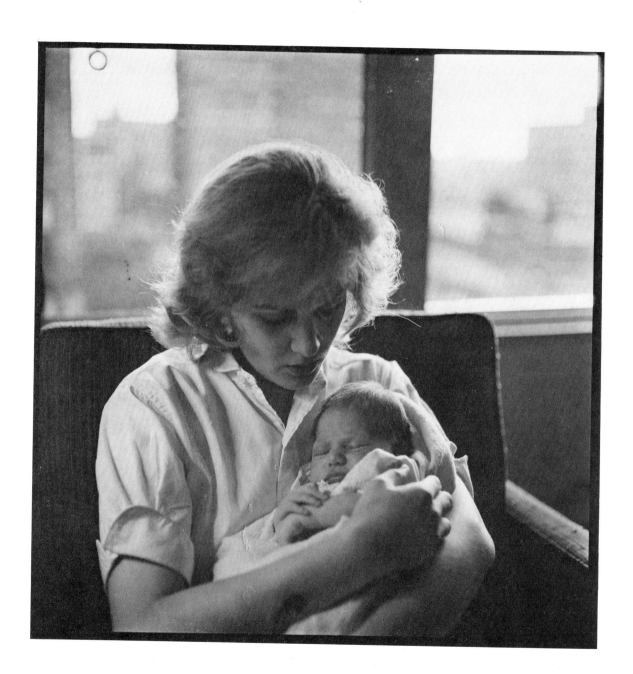

loved to think about having a family. When Sally grew up, she met Ted. They planned to get married. One of their nicest plans was all about the joy of having their own children. After they were married, they thought, ''Oh good, now at last we can have our baby.'' But a long time passed, and Sally did not become pregnant. The doctor then told them that something was wrong; they couldn't have their own baby. At first Sally cried. All her life she had wanted a family! Ted was disappointed too.

After a while, they decided that the Lord wanted them to be parents to somebody who had not been born to them. They were very excited and happy. ''Let's ask the Lord to choose the special baby who should be a part of our family. We will adopt a baby!''

They knew that there were babies and children who needed new families. Being a mother or father means that you say, ''Yes, I choose to care for and love this child as my own. I name this child as mine.'' Sally and Ted had to wait a long time before they could adopt a baby. But finally Sally held her adopted baby close in her arms. She whispered, ''Oh, how I have longed for you. Just you.'' Ted was overjoyed. His family was growing. ''Our house was made for at least three children,'' he said. ''I hope that the Lord lets us have a big family.''

Adoption is a way of choosing to help babies or children who need a new family for some reason. Some of you who read this book may be adopted,

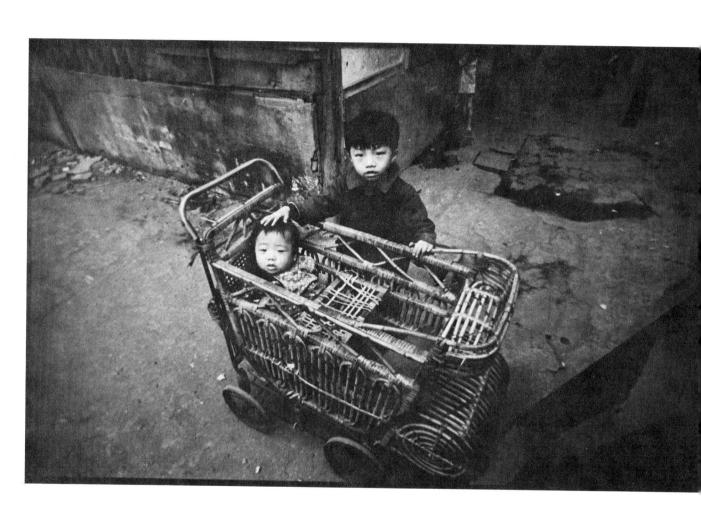

chosen to be your parents' very own child. Or maybe one of your brothers or sisters was adopted. Maybe you can remember the wonderful day when the new family member came home.

Every person in the world is special. When someone needs extra care, we must help to make things right and good.

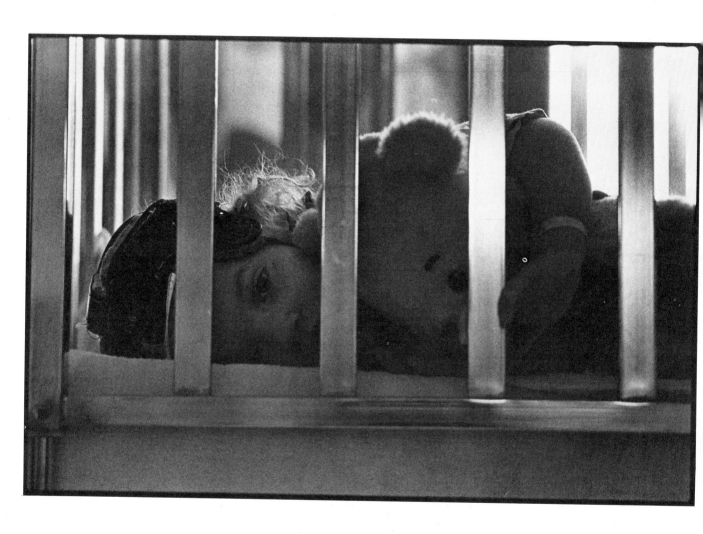

6
When Something Goes Wrong

Once upon a time there was a real boy. He had won a special prize. He was to have a trip in a helicopter. On the day before the ride, he was rushed to the hospital because he was sick. The little boy got better, but to his bitter disappointment, he had missed the ride.

Things can go wrong in your body even before you are born. The problem here is that sometimes this affects the part of the body that is being made on that day. The real boy missed his ride, but some babies miss a day of growth and development on a day when a particular part of their body is being formed.

Perhaps something happened, for example, the day that the roof of your mouth was being formed. It's strange, but if you missed that day's progress, you could be born with a hole in the roof of your mouth.

73

This is called a cleft palate. You would then need an operation to fix it up when you were older.

That is not so bad. But sometimes something disturbs a baby the day its arm bud makes a hand, or something else really important to its body. If you missed that day of development, then you would never have your hand. This is something hard to live with. If you are reading or hearing this book and you were born with everything perfectly made, you should be thankful. Some of you will read the book and think, ''That is the story of when I was a baby. That is why I had something wrong when I was born.''

It is good to remember that nobody in this world is perfect anyway. Some problems just *show* more than others. Nothing can change the fact that you are a person, important, and made with the same purpose as anybody else. We all *do* different things in life anyway. It is who we *are* that matters. It also matters that we are members of God's family.

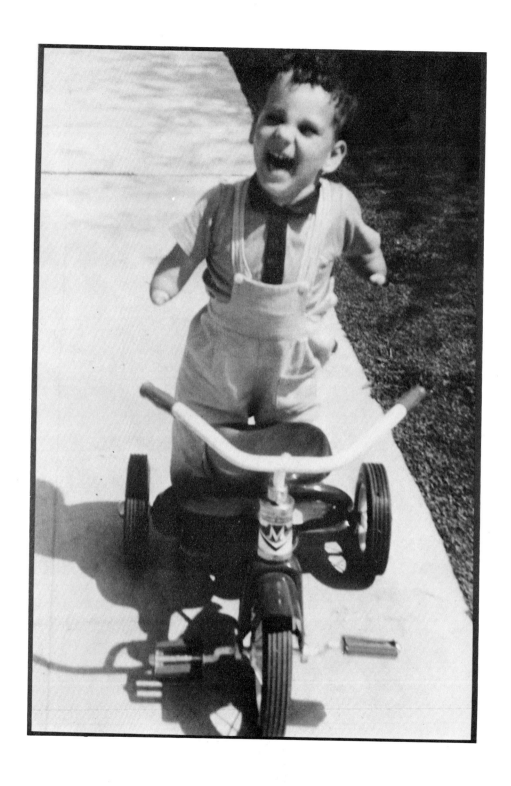

Craig's Story

Perhaps I can give you a better idea of what I mean by telling you about several friends of mine. I know a boy named Craig. As you can see in this picture, when he was an unborn baby, his arms did not develop as they should. Also, one leg was missing. Sometimes he felt angry and frustrated when he tried to do things. Sometimes he was left out of games other children could play. These experiences were difficult for him.

His aunt was a hospital worker called an occupational therapist. She helped people learn to do things even if something had gone wrong with their bodies. She made little artificial arms for Craig when he was still a baby. Later he could play with toys and feed himself. He had fun like any other toddler. When he was old enough, he went to school just like anybody else. His friends thought he was clever, because he could draw and write with his special hands. He was a good friend to have. He had lots of ideas for games. His ideas were clever, because he was used to thinking things out when it was hard.

Now that Craig is grown up, he has finished college and is at a theological seminary. That means he is studying the Bible so that he can help people and teach them the truth of the Bible. He will be able to help people when they are sad, because he has had hard times, too, with his handicap. He knows that different kinds of things can go wrong in people's lives, but he also knows how God helps us even when our lives aren't perfect. There is not one person in this whole world who is as perfect as he would like to be.

One thing that can happen to a baby about this age is especially hard. Sometimes as the brain is being formed, something goes wrong. So when the baby is born, he or she may look fine, but there is a hidden handicap.

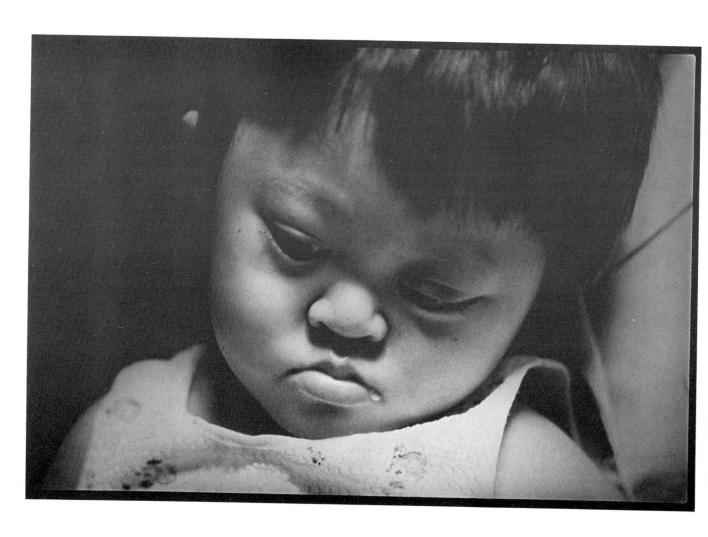

Alice's Story

Alice looked like any other baby when she was born. But soon her mother noticed that she didn't suck her milk very well. She didn't smile or laugh like her sister Emily had when she was several weeks old. She didn't reach for toys.

Alice had a mother, father, and a big sister in her family. They loved their new baby. Emily liked to hold her, and she would rock her in the rocking chair. The mother liked to sing to her new daughter.

The doctor told them that there was something wrong with their baby. He told them that something had gone wrong with Alice's brain while she was being made. She was mentally retarded.

Alice's parents were terribly sad when they heard this news. They could see that their little girl was beautiful. It was not good that she would miss being able to do as much as other people can all their lives. Parents are happy to see their children strong and well. Alice's parents knew that they would have to work harder to care for her. They knew that it would be hard for Alice, too.

They went to talk to a Christian friend about it. The mother said, "Why did this have to happen to Alice?"

Their friend explained that the whole world had

been ruined when Adam and Eve sinned. God hadn't wanted children to be born handicapped or pain, or fighting, or death. He didn't want people to be hungry or to be in wars. He had so wanted the world to be good.

But God planned a way for the world to be made new again. That time hasn't come yet. Alice's parents wished that the time had come for it to be fixed up. They wanted to see Alice develop just like Emily had. They were glad, though, that Jesus had promised us that he is coming back again. Then, when the world is made new as he promised, everything will be good again. They knew that Alice would be perfectly okay then. They knew that God thought she was as precious and special a person as anybody else. Meanwhile, they knew that the Lord would help them and their Alice in life *right now*, too. God cared that their situation was difficult.

Alice's parents wanted to do all that they could for her. But they weren't sure *what* to do. Then they met a family with a child who was mentally retarded, too. His name was Tim and he was five. Tim's whole family was a help to Alice's family. As they explained quite a lot about Tim, Alice's mother and father felt better. They did not feel so alone with their problems anymore. The families often visited each other after that. They prayed together and helped each other.

I hope that *you* were all okay in those weeks when you were only tiny and you were growing in the womb. If you were made without anything going wrong at all, that is good. But some people *do* have something wrong, either in themselves or in their family. That is why when we think about babies, we have to think about those who have something wrong as well as those who are fine.

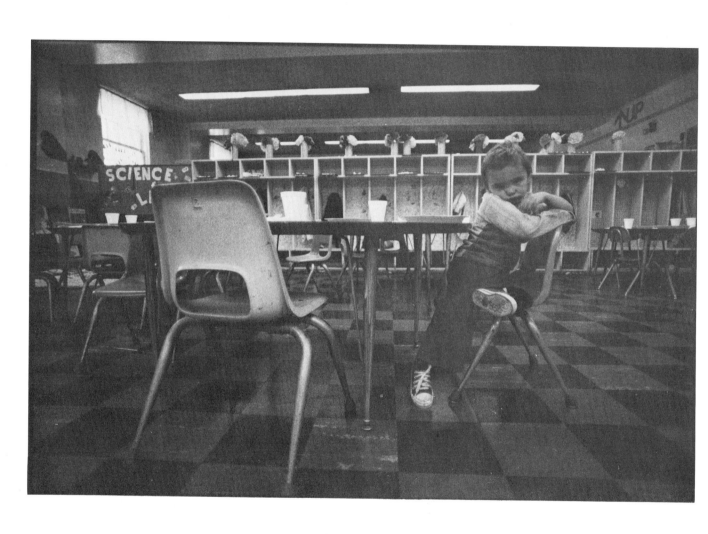

Tim's Story

Tim's story is an interesting one.

When he was born, the doctor said he had something wrong. He had Down's syndrome, and that meant he would look different. He would be mentally retarded, and he would learn slowly.

When he was tiny, Tim hadn't looked around much. So his parents bought lots of colorful toys, and his mother would swing them back and forth in front of him. One day he started following the toys with his eyes. When he was older, he started smiling. Later on, he laughed.

Tim didn't make any sounds like "da-da-da." So Tim's mother talked to him a lot. She sang him songs. That was important to Tim. But still he was quiet. Tim's mother propped him up and moved his arms and legs around. He needed help to make his muscles strong. She put him where he could see his family. Of course, this special care took a lot of time. When Tim's dad came home from work, he would carry Tim around on his back. Tim liked his dad's deep voice.

One day, much later, Tim sat up for the first time. The whole family clapped and laughed. They all loved Tim extra specially because he needed their help such a lot. They were thrilled every time he

85

learned something new.

When Tim was about a year old, he finally crawled around. He had lots of fun getting into everything!

Tim's big brother Peter liked to help Tim "walk." He would hold on to Tim's hands and walk him around the room. Tim was getting really strong now. He even learned to walk by himself when he was about two years old. That was an exciting day! Tim's father liked to make cakes. He made a big one to celebrate that day. They let Tim's big brother Peter invite in all of his friends. Peter had helped Tim such a lot. He was proud of his baby brother.

Tim did naughty things, too. He once took out all the ashes from the fireplace when the fire wasn't burning. He threw them all over the room. What a mess! The family helped clean up.

Tim's parents were glad when Tim learned what no meant. That was important.

One day something funny happened. Tim had never fed himself. He liked his food, but he never put it in his own mouth. Just before supper one day Peter suddenly noticed that Timmy had eaten all the cat's dinner from the cat dish.

"Oh no," groaned his mother. "He'll get sick." She worried about it, but afterwards she was pleased. Tim really was getting to be more like any other toddler. After that, she put Tim's food on his high-chair tray. He wasn't very good at feeding himself. Food got in his eyes and nose. He practically needed a bath after every meal! But soon he got better at it.

When Tim was three and a half, he was a happy little boy. He couldn't ride a tricycle. He couldn't talk yet. But he had learned how to go to the toilet. Everybody in the family had to help Tim learn this. It was harder for him to learn than it usually is.

The family had let Tim come to the bathroom and see them use the toilet. Tim liked to copy them. Everybody would say, ''Hurrah for you, Tim.'' Tim would smile and smile. Of course, it was a nuisance for the family, too. Tim made a lot of puddles all over the house. He didn't like the feel of wet pants, so his mother or father would get him dry again right away. Finally Tim learned to wait until he could get to the bathroom. He was funny. He couldn't talk yet, so guess how he told the others that he wanted to go? He would pull down his pants and stand there! Then somebody would rush him off to the bathroom.

Peter pretended that Tim wasn't his brother when Tim did that in the middle of the supermarket!

When Tim was nearly four, he ''talked'' his own funny mixed-up sounds, even though they had no meaning. He liked to play with the other neighborhood children in his yard.

When Tim's parents decided that he was ready for school, Tim entered a kindergarten class. He loved the slide. He liked painting pictures.

The other children liked playing with Tim. He was a good friend to them. They didn't mind that he couldn't talk yet. Tim liked school so much that he would cry when it was time to go home.

Tim found it hard that no one could understand what he wanted. He still couldn't talk. Sometimes he would get red in the face with anger, and he would kick. Talking is one of the best things we can do. Imagine if you couldn't ever *tell* anybody anything at all.

Then Tim started trying to copy the things his family said. They were careful to say "bus," "car," or "cow" when they drove past one. At home they would say "drink" or "book." Tim became interested in picture books. He sat up on his dad's lap and tried to copy the words by the pictures. The family was excited when Tim could start to talk. Tim would say, "muk, muk" for milk, then "be..d, be..d" for bread.

At last Tim was really talking. He could say, "gimme dwink," "ba..dog" (bad dog).

Tim went to Sunday School. He liked the singing. He had a special song that he would clap and sing. His teacher played it every week for the children: "Praise Him, praise Him, all you little children."

The people at church knew that it was hard work for Tim's family. They knew that his mother had to teach Tim a lot of things most children learn quickly. So other families would have Tim over to play some days. Tim liked visiting his church friends. Then Tim's parents could go shopping or take Peter out somewhere more easily.

Twice a year Tim's friends had him come and stay for a whole week. That way Tim's mother and father and Peter could have fun doing things that their little Tim couldn't manage. Sometimes they went on bike trips with camping gear. Once they went skiing.

Tim's family loved him a lot. They enjoyed him. He was fun and funny. Tim was so loving, and he always wore a smile. They would have never traded Tim in for anybody else. Tim needed them more than most children would. Sometimes Tim's mother would sigh, "I wish that Jesus would come back now. Then I could see Tim all perfect. I wouldn't have to wait anymore. That day will be so special for Tim."

His father sometimes said, "It will be my happiest day to see my little son made perfect. It will be wonderful to have a good talk together! I love Tim so much! But I am happy that Tim has been able to learn such a lot even though he is handicapped. And I am thankful that he is such a kind, thoughtful boy. God has been good to us all. He has helped us have good ideas, and he has answered prayers in many ways."

Maybe some children in your family, neighborhood, school, or church need your love and help in a special way. Think of ways that you can do nice things for them or help them. When will you do it?

All of us have things go wrong one way or another. We all need each other's help at different times. And each one of us is a special, separate person that matters to God. He knows our name, he loves us, and he will be our best helper right through our entire life.

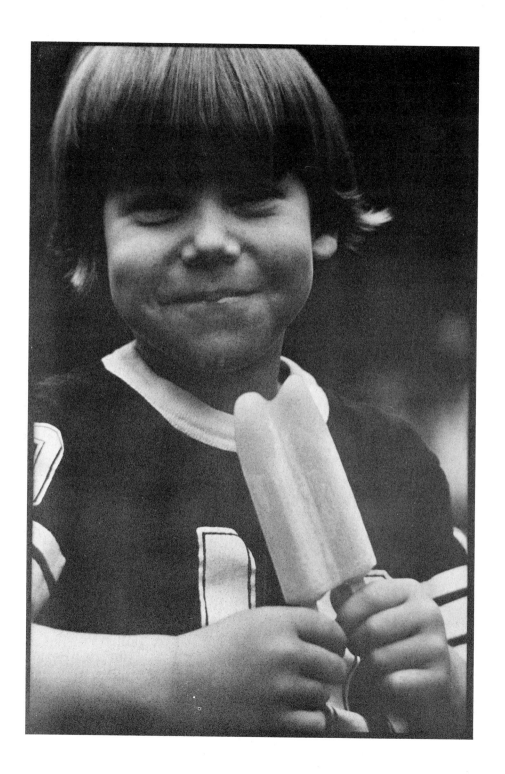

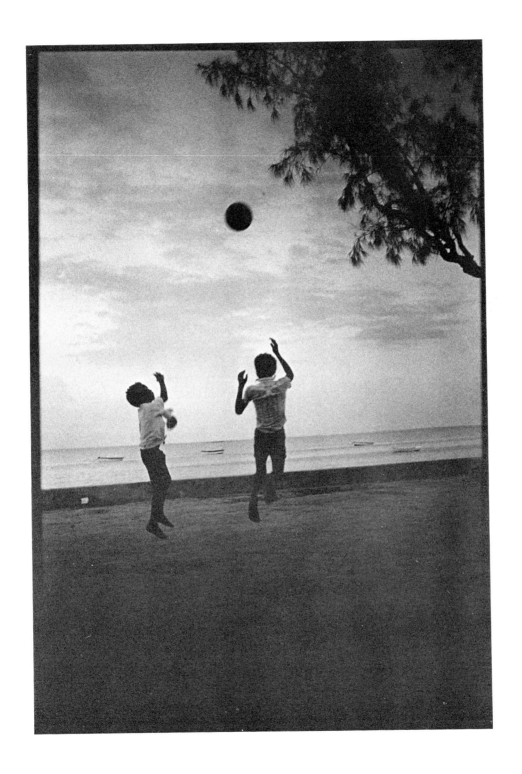

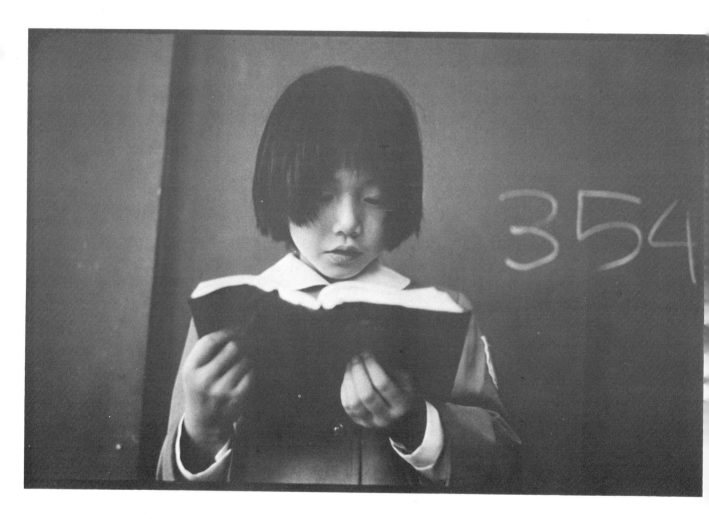

Publisher's Note

Something Beautiful From God has sought to capture the mystery and worth of God's priceless gift of life. The different elements which make up the book—the text, design, photography, printing—all were selected with this goal in mind.

As the publisher, we would like to express our special thanks to those who made this not only a book, but a work of art . . .

To Susan Schaeffer Macaulay for the vision to write a book filled with wonder and compassion . . .

To Ray Cioni and his studio, The Cioni Artworks, for translating the written word into a moving visual experience . . .

To Ron Seymour for providing the black and white photography—photography which so beautifully portrays the innocence and reality of childhood . . .

To *Parents* magazine for graciously providing the in-the-womb photography by Manus Huller—photography which captures the miracle of life-before-birth as no illustration or diagram ever could . . .

To the printer, Lithocolor Press, for faithfully reproducing all of these elements in printed form.